FOOD FOR THE JOURNEY TO "I AM"

Harvest of Healing, LLC

Publishing assistance by BookCrafters, Parker, Colorado.

www.bookcrafters.net

Trusting and Believing have been contaminated by the desire to understand.

This Book is dedicated to all
Current and future generations of Spiritual Royals
Who will continue to bring forth Ancient Customs
Resulting in the opportunity to live life in The Way of I AM.

TABLE OF CONTENTS

FOOD FOR THE JOURNEY TO "I AM"

UNTANGLING THE MYTHS OF FOOD AND EXERCISE

The information I share is by no means a prescription for any form of cure to any ailment, sickness or disease. What is shared are results and observances from the experiences I encountered through years of a journey to regain my health, and what has been found within Scripture to back up some of those discoveries. It is up to each individual to decide in what order and to what degree they desire to implement the Spiritual Royal lifestyle.

INTRODUCTION

This book is an initial effort to summon those who qualify through a means of genetics to discover and implement the Ancient Ways referred to in Scripture. The food suggestions herein are not a prescription or promise for relief of any disease, sickness or diagnosis. I am not a physician and will not make any claim that what is shared or that copying my personal experience will cure anyone. Curing someone is God's job. Attempting to discover what was lost long ago when it comes to having the ability to not only heal myself but provide insight to others for their health journey has proven to be time consuming and at times costly. There is still much more to discover and learn. What I share is just a fraction of what will continue to come forth.

Food and food choices are in desperate need of some fine-tuning. Surprisingly, foods that appear healthy and you think should be healthy are not always the case for a Spiritual Royal who is attempting to elevate the electrical charge within the Wheels and blood cells.

Each person's body will need a little different measure of what is set forth in these pages. Some will have a quick response internally and for some it will take longer. Every "body" is different. As the food suggestions are implemented the body can have any number of reactions, from headaches, fatigue, insomnia, flu-like symptoms to elevated emotions. The body has strange responses when you decide to change its routine and clean it out.

Food selection is not the only component to the Ancient Ways that needs restored; customs, social interactions and overall lifestyle will have adjustments as well. Recovery of the way life was lived by those once called Wise Women or Wise Men takes time when there are no known written instructions for that lifestyle other than Scripture. If you are up for the challenge of obtaining a status that graduates a person into "Eternal Life", then this is where you start.

John 4:14: *But whoever drinks from the water that I will give him will never get thirsty again – ever! In fact, the water I will give him will become a well of water springing up within him for eternal life.* (HCS)

This book is in no way an attempt to get everyone on a bandwagon of a certain diet plan in hopes of correcting any specific ailment. What is brought forth is what Scripture teaches about food selections and my own personal journey through the process of changing my food selections to line up with what Scripture teaches in order to cause transformation within the blood cells; the transformation that erases inherited genetic imprints for disease; and the benefits and challenges I experienced. It is my hope to initiate a change in the lifestyle humans have come to accept that has resulted in numerous health disturbances. This new way of sustaining life through food and activity

4

is not meant to be a temporary fix but what should be implemented from this day forward that will walk mankind into the Ancient Ways foretold of in Scripture. I'm on my way to living as a *Spiritual Royal*.

FROM THE INSIDE OUT

Mankind has evolved into a position of being focused on what is externally good, seemingly beneficial, perfect, beautiful or sin-free. Humans mold, shape, cut and form their bodies in all different ways and in all areas of the body. Is this all an attempt to impress or catch the eye of someone or something important? Who are we here on this earth to impress? I agree that proper dress or fashion and hygiene are a must. Please do not go to that public meeting with unattended hair or teeth that lack being brushed.

I doubt the total dollar amount spent on surgeries, cosmetics, sports or recreational exercise to modify the physical body, prescription medications to eliminate blemishes or other noticeable so called defects, is even calculable. Why do humans apply so much money and time into something that can and will alter when the proper foods are eaten and balanced activity is adopted? An obvious answer would be because we were never taught such a thing was possible. Many of the attempts people make to acquire that beauty (attractive or handsome) are only temporary. Beauty is fleeting is the old saying. Why go to all the extra fuss if altering food choice can develop into an exterior beauty?

When you become familiar with Scripture and follow the general story lines, noting how certain person's were addressed when being greeted or described by the prophets, you begin to recognize there was a beauty attached to a specific group of people. Some of these people, who were given this description of beauty, fair complexion or blue eyed, were also noted as choosing a meal of vegetables, fruits and grains over meats. This raises a question in my mind as to whether our food choices, and those of our ancestors, have had a part to play in the existing hair color, eye color or even skin pigmentation differences evident today. What I have witnessed is when a diet switches from one particular food group that was eaten regularly to a totally different category of foods (meats to vegetables), the hair color begins to change shades. Of course this is over an extended period of time, not just a one-week transition. This creates a fascinating line of thought, if nothing else.

Our focus, attention and efforts are to be directed to the interior. This is not just a reference to our opinions, emotions and how we speak to someone which all has value but what Scripture is talking about is the interior health and function of the physical body. Food choices, exercise choices, quality of the sounds we listen to daily (music or other 'noise') all have a measure of effect upon our interior health and environment.

Most have come to accept that God is described as light, power and/or energy and strength so would it not make sense that our focus should be on our internal ability to generate light, power and energy? We are "made in His image" although it would be impossible to physically look like God on the exterior. With the proper power (electrical connection or conduction), the physical body will react and respond as it was designed to. Emotions can be properly dealt with and not become stuck in our cells, tissues and thoughts or brain tissues; the Wheels (batteries) along our spine, often identified as chakras, stay charged up, our body is healthy and life all around in general just works better. We graduate into a position of being able to give off light, a trait connected to the descriptions of God. With that light on the inside, a person will display a beauty. What's on the inside will begin to reflect through to the exterior altering the many traits people identify each other by.

1 John 1:7: *But if we walk in the light as He Himself is in the light, we have fellowship with one another, and the blood of Jesus His Son cleanses us from all sin.* (HCS)

1 John 5:6-8: *Jesus Christ – He is the One who came by water and blood, not by water only, but by water and by blood. And the Spirit is the One who testifies, because the Spirit is the truth. For there are three that testify: the Spirit, the water, and the blood – and these three are in agreement.* (HCS)

A NEW DIRECTION

II Chronicles 29:5-9: He said to them, "Hear me, Levites. Consecrate yourselves now and consecrate the temple of Yahweh, the God of your ancestors. Remove everything impure from the holy place. For our fathers were unfaithful and did what is evil in the sight of the Lord our God. They abandoned Him, turned their faces away from the Lord's tabernacle, and turned their backs on Him. They also closed the doors of the portico, extinguished the lamps, did not burn incense, and did not offer burnt offerings in the holy place of the God of Israel. Therefore, the wrath of the Lord was on Judah (praise) and Jerusalem (peace), and He made them an object of terror, horror, and mockery, as you see with your own eyes. Our fathers fell by the sword, and our sons, our daughters, and our wives are in captivity because of this. It is in my heart now to make a covenant with Yahweh, the God of Israel so that His burning anger may turn away from us. My sons, don't be negligent now, for the Lord has chosen you to stand in His presence, to serve Him, and to be His ministers and burners of incense." (HCS) (Inserts added)

These verses are a call to a specific group of people, to clean up their eating habits (and other harmful practices) that will result in clearing out harmful and potentially deadly issues from happening inside the body (temple).

The descriptive terms used are reference to the internal mechanisms of the physical body. The acts of this people group will assist others in their journey to clean their own bodily temples (houses). Bottom line is, we must clean up our "temple" (body) or the road many are currently traveling will likely become a slippery slope that leads to an uncomfortable trip to the cemetery.

ON THE JOURNEY

I can only speak from my personal experience and I have no _formal_ training when it comes to the body functions and nutrition. I share what I have found to be beneficial and what became hindering.

Many foods can be processed through the digestive system with no known (or noticed) side effects or discomfort but that does not mean those foods do not have a negative affect on the cells or the amount of Wheel electricity it takes to process them. The cells pick up on the messages encoded in the food, the vibrations, and the cells will either be energized or drained by those vibrations. Many foods that are common today have been through some form of processing that can deplete or alter the nutritional content and there are some foods that do not qualify as beneficial until some form of preparation is complete. Some foods common to us today should not be eaten at all, even though they are approved by the regulatory board(s) that put a stamp on what they qualify as food. I am not only referencing the processed meats, there are some items within the fresh produce section of your local grocery store that should be avoided. I am not familiar with the history of where some of the avoid items originated but most likely they were the result of an accidental cross-contamination, experiment or a bright idea. God is the originator of foods and when humans put their hand in the mix and alter the original, the altered food can become disastrous for the physical body. We are a species that has become successful at killing our own kind.

The food guidelines for a *Spiritual Royal* are not easy to follow, especially in the times we currently live. As time moves forward and the word gets out, the selections of food for the *Spiritual Royal* will expand.

LIFE IS IN THE WHEELS

The goal for a *Spiritual Royal* is to have all electrical centers (Wheels) healthy and working properly. Symptoms and ultimately disease can often be the result of failing or hindered electrical charge of the Wheel(s). When the Wheels are functioning and healthy the systems that do their work in the body are operating well, health is prosperous, not stressed.

There is an abundance of Internet and published information on the Chakra (Sanskrit for Wheel) system. I invite you to review some of that information and become familiar with how the specific color of a food coincides with a specific Wheel. A color code system was attached to the Wheels system for ease in identification. Verses within the book of Ezekiel describe the colors by reference to a mineral stone. They lacked the color pallet in Biblical times so they referenced color according to what they were familiar with in nature. Using a chart of the Wheels and their respective colors will assist in determining which food(s) may be necessary in response to a symptom the body experiences.

What the current chakra charts and food selections do not contain are foods that can cause harm or cancel out the beneficial food you eat, or the activity you may do

13

that can hinder recharge of the Wheel. Just because a food has a coordinating color does not necessarily mean it will charge the Wheel. Also, there are foods outside of the food color chart that can cancel out all of your effort to charge the Wheels. There are various accepted styles of exercise that can deplete the Wheels or hinder the recharge.

The goal is to implement a strategy that helps you avoid some of the foods and exercises that can cause a set back when you are attempting to recharge the Wheels. Some of the "avoid foods" may not have to always be excluded after the Wheels are fully charged and functioning, although just as one would periodically charge a cell phone, the Wheels must be recharged periodically as well. The pattern of recharge would be solely dependent upon what the individual has encountered and what their daily habits are. Strenuous physical activity may cause that individual's Wheels to drain their energy faster than one who has a generally balanced level of activity. After the general concept of use and recharge is identified within the individual, just like use of your cell phone, there will be signs or symptoms within the body that remind you a recharge is necessary. The quicker you drain the Wheels of their charge, the quicker you will need to take time to recharge.

Ideas on how to avoid those foods that can set you back are shared in general categories in the Topics that follow. You want to avoid the two steps forward, one step back process or you could end up on a very long journey through transition. The food restrictions that assist in charging

Wheels is challenging enough so avoiding a back slide is key. Once the Wheels are healthy and fully charged, it not only ushers in vitality and abundant life to the body but also brings forth a component of the *Spiritual Royal* status. From this point it is acts of maintaining the health and charge of the Wheels through food and activity versus effort to regain the necessary charge.

I found that Wheels like for you to keep them warm. Being cold uses the charge in the Wheel when you shiver as an act to stay warm. Dress warm and take warm baths or showers. Sitting in a tub of warm-hot water of an evening acts as a benefit for the Wheel activity. The body does a lot of house cleaning while you sleep so happy, warm Wheels is a benefit to those housekeeping chores going on during your sleep.

Many of the foods can be consumed raw, steamed or cooked. If you choose to eat raw foods, warm the stomach prior to beginning your meal and during the meal. Drink a hot cup of brewed chicory root or hot water with cut fresh ginger and a squeeze of lemon juice. It is common practice to preheat an oven before you put food in it to bake, why wouldn't the same concept apply to the stomach?

WORKING WITH ENERGY

There are lifestyle choices that need change before the Ancient Ways become evident; food and physical activity all need alterations. Humans abuse the physical body and expect God to repair it. This may seem shocking but God does not work for the medical industry or at the gym down the street.

II Kings 1:6: *They replied, "A man came to meet us and said, 'Go back to the king who sent you and declare to him: This is what the Lord says: Is it because there is no God in Israel that you're sending these men to inquire of Baal-zebub, the god of Ekron? Therefore, you will not get up from your sickbed – you will certainly die.'"* (HCS) (Ekron: uproot; barrenness).

God works much differently than what has been adopted by a means of medical science and consulting the sources outside of God Himself can result in a disastrous situation. A dose of God's preventative ways will result in a huge benefit.

There is true natural energy and conjured up energy. Some might claim the response (rush or energized) to strenuous exercise is natural, which is true, in part. An individual can force their body into a specific state or reaction. This is not a natural process but a manipulated process.

Three categories of energy to consider: Natural production of energy through the cells and various processes of the body; the Heaven Energy provided by God; and an energy produced by stimulation of the nervous system as one would get through caffeine, energy drinks, strenuous exercise or stimulation of the meridians (electrical highways in the body).

Two of the expressions of physical energy can appear the same yet have a different source of influence, natural or stimulated. The same rings true for Spiritual energy. A person can appear to have a connection with the Heaven Energy source(s) when actually they have a conjured up energy at work. These are situations to be cautious of when working with or seeking the guidance from one who claims expertise in energy therapies. In order to receive something permanent, you want the genuine, not a counterfeit that is temporary.

Colossians 1:29: *I labor for this, striving with His strength that works powerfully in me.* (KJV)

Looking through a more Scientific lens, activities that have taken place, or the lack of specific activities, has caused the Heaven Energy we need here on Earth to deplete; the battery charge required for the Wheels in the physical body fades and nature becomes stressed. The actions that have resulted in the depleted charge has been no one's fault but humanity itself. What needs to take place is for humanity to correct their harmful habits and get their Wheels recharged, which not only helps their physical health but will begin to aid the planet in its regeneration to vitality.

GENETICS

Scriptures reference different people groups; people from differing regions or customs, not necessarily pointing to a religious separation. When Scripture was written some regions did represent variations in religious practices and beliefs but not always. Most every religion is accessible all over the world today so in order to apply these Scripture references in a context useful for today, we will focus on genetic factors or ethnic backgrounds. The bloodline of Abraham, Isaac and Jacob is mentioned with specifics.

Isaiah 41:8-10: *But you, Israel, My servant, Jacob, whom I have chosen, descendant of Abraham, My Friend I brought you from the ends of the earth and called you from its farthest corners. I said to you: You are My servant; I have chosen you and not rejected you. Do not fear, for I am with you; do not be afraid, for I am your God. I will strengthen you; I will help you; I will hold on to you with My righteous right hand.* (HCS)

There are also references to certain persons being pointed out as a "Hebrew" which indicates a Hebrew had specific physical features that were different from the rest of the crowd. Something about their physical appearance was evident and noticed even though they dressed in long flowing clothes of linen.

Exodus 2:5-6: *Pharaoh's daughter went down to bathe at the Nile while her servant girls walked along the riverbank. Seeing the basket among the reeds, she sent her slave girl to get it. When she opened it, she saw the child – a little boy, crying. She felt sorry for him and said, "This is one of the Hebrew boys."* (HCS)

Sticking with the thought of appearing "different", whether you are familiar with the stories in Scripture or not, it points to genetics. I'm going to step out on a limb here and certainly have no form of evidence but I think the genetic reference could indicate that people from the genetic line of "Abraham, Isaac and Jacob" will have a greater success rate when it comes to <u>completing</u> the steps of transformation involved in order to qualify as a *Spiritual Royal*. Why? There must be some genetic code that allows the transformation process to progress forward (I don't want to say "more easily" because this is not easy no matter how you slice it) where in other ethnic or genetic groups it may be more challenging or take more time. This could also be in part due to the stress experienced by and the eating habits of ancestors. One ethnic group may have more ancestors that ate foods not compatible to Wheel health and vitality versus another ethnic group of ancestors who ate more Wheel friendly foods. Honestly, all I can go by is what is referenced in Scripture. We will come to know more as time moves forward.

AGE LIMITS

<u>I Chronicles 23:3-5</u>: The Levites 30 years old or more were counted; the total number of men was 38,000 by headcount. Of these, David said, "24,000 are to be in charge of the work on the Lord's temple, 6,000 are to be officers and judges, 4,000 are to be gatekeepers, and 4,000 are to praise the Lord with instruments that I have made for worship." (HCS)

The status of a *Spiritual Royal* will not be obtainable to anyone under the age of 30 years old. This coincides with the verses in I Chronicles and with the experiences Jesus had leading up to the crucifixion. His sufferings exhibit an example of the processes the body will go through when harmful debris are being escorted out of the cells (and tissues); it can cause some discomforts and varying symptoms.

It is always beneficial to instill proper eating habits to your children and it will certainly help them in the long run especially when they decide to have children of their own. Good childhood eating habits will be a jump-start for them when they are of the age to progress forward to a *Spiritual Royal.*

HOW HARD IS IT?

Obtaining and maintaining the status of a *Spiritual Royal* is quite challenging in the world we live in today. First, in order to obtain the status of what I have selected to call a *Spiritual Royal*, an individual must complete the processes required to eliminate harmful frequencies inside the cells in their body (mainly the blood). Second, foods that provide fuel for the Wheels so they can recharge and recover is a must. It may feel like you have few options when it comes to food but it will inspire your creative side when it comes time to prepare dinner.

The Wheels must work to aid the cells in eliminating the harmful imprints they hold (aka the Sin). An individual may be born with a greater measure of *Spiritual Royal* genetics but to date, everyone needs to clean out the toxic debris inside the cells to move toward a classification of *Spiritual Royal*. A more in depth description of the frequencies inside cells and how they get there can be found in the book: *From AntiChrist to "I AM"* published Spring 2022.

During the processes required that ultimately erase the harmful frequencies, the *Spiritual Royal* food selections should be gradually implemented, not to overwhelm the body yet giving the body the opportunity to have the ability to make use of the beneficial food and nutrients.

Keep in mind, there are negative and positives to everything and that applies to foods as well. The body does not operate well, and will eventually develop symptoms or disease, when intake of the negative foods outweighs the intake of the positive ones. For this concept to be easier followed, think of food as being the money in your bank account. When the proper Spirit (beneficial) foods are eaten you make a deposit; and when Flesh (harmful) foods are eaten there is a withdrawal. Neutral foods have no affect on the account balance but when the Wheel bank account is overdrawn, there will be penalties and fines (sickness, fatigue, insomnia, etc.) It's also like adding low-grade fuel to a fancy new Ferrari, it will not run well and eventually there will be a mechanic's bill to pay.

Many have lived their life on a Standard American Diet so this new way of choosing foods and eliminating many of the standard foods we've grown accustom to can be overwhelming. The USDA approved food pyramid needs to be erased when you are working towards and maintaining the level and lifestyle of *Spiritual Royal.* Take baby steps while also moving forward to obtain the end goal.

There will be times when the body seems to continually remind you that it wants the food it became accustomed to having. Food choices or cravings seem to be recorded inside the cells and can often scream at us that we "want chocolate" (or whatever your food of choice is). These pre-recorded choices can be erased or recorded over, it just takes some time. The body will eventually shift and not continually crave those old favorites. Part of the craving is engrained in the brain and as you progress through the new food choices, the brain will adjust. Those engrained thoughts of "If Grandma and Momma said it is good for you, isn't it good for you?" will fade. Do the best you can to not waiver from the straight and narrow but when you do, get back on track as soon as possible.

THAT'S WAY TOO MUCH

Having been programmed to "clean your plate" from the time we become big enough to hold a spoon has not resulted in much benefit. The "clean your plate" thought pattern should be erased. Eat what you need, when you feel full, stop eating. There is no benefit in stressing the body to process more food than what is necessary. Americans love the "super size" concept but there is a need to consider what that super size may be doing to the electrical activity required to process it (or what it may be doing to the waistline).

Try not to stress eat. Eating under stressful times is borne out of habit to attempt to relieve a nagging *E-motion.* If you must have something, eat a carrot, cucumber or piece of fruit. You want to avoid overworking the Wheels when it is not necessary.

DINNER BELLS

Eat when the body tells you it is hungry. School schedules and work schedules have caused the habit of eating when the clock strikes "lunch hour", whatever time that is for you. If we are not hungry and yet we eat a full meal, it adds a burden to the digestive system and process. Let the internal systems of the body do the talking. They are telling you when they are ready for the next meal, and so on. Somewhere along the line people forgot how to listen to the internal voice.

RELAX INTO IT

Take time for reflection or meditation; be thankful that the body is healthy and has the ability to be healthy; you might envision a cleansing process or light sweeping through your body, which brings restoration. Worry is not a beneficial tool to carry around and can quickly drain the Wheels. The mind is a powerful machine and the body will follow your thoughts.

Matthew 6:33-34: *But seek first the kingdom of God and His righteousness, and all these things will be provided for you. Therefore don't worry about tomorrow because tomorrow will worry about itself. Each day has enough trouble of its own.* (HCS)

ORGANIC IS A MUST

Eat clean organic fruits, vegetables and whole grains, nothing processed or fortified. Clean foods are much easier for the digestive system to process and therefore take less of your Wheel energy. Chemically treated foods create a negative response and would cancel out any Wheel charge value in the food nutritionally (I'm speaking energetically here).

Put foods under a black light and observe the light that is given off by an organic (no chemical treatment) product versus a chemically treated product. We need foods with good "light" in them for the cells to be healthy and Wheels to charge. I saw a video a few years ago that was part of a class I was taking online and it shared the results of an experiment done on the light/colors produced by foods and supplements. Foods that give off the most energy/color is what the body needs. I haven't researched to see if other videos of this type exist in a general web search but most likely they do.

TAKE A BREATH

Learn to belly breath. God breathed into Adam's nostrils and there was <u>life</u>. Take air in through the nose, expand and fill the belly and chest, release the air through the mouth to expel toxins. This is beneficial for the lungs and circulation, and your blood will thank you for the oxygen! Take 3 or 4 slow belly breaths and rest. Do this however often you feel necessary throughout the day. The breath creates a movement inside the body. It is also a form of praise. ("Let everything that has breath praise the Lord.")

Like the wind that moves the clouds or waters; that fans the flames of a fire or moves the dirt and dust of the ground, that same concept is necessary for the interior of the physical body. Those who live at high altitudes may need to work at the breathing a little more than those at sea level.

TIME FOR RECESS

I cannot say that I thought recess was the best part of elementary school. I saw no good reason in standing outside in the freezing cold! Although, it was nice to take a break from the desk and those exercises for the brain held within the pages of textbooks.

It is beneficial to spend some time outdoors in a quiet surrounding. If possible, sit and soak up some rays from the sun (with a hat covering your head). Your body needs refreshment, time away from the desk or the mop and broom, whatever your daily routine activity is. The Earth herself will enjoy your company and the suit you reside in called the body, will thank you.

I WANT TO GO!

Traveling in this day and age will be extremely challenging simply because restaurant foods are not always *Spiritual Royal* friendly. Salad with no dressing and a sweet potato with a dollop of <u>real</u> butter might be your only options. In time, some restaurants and cafes will become aware of the up and coming ways of food selections and make a shift towards better cell-friendly choices. Until then, if you must travel, a grocery store may be your best option for something edible.

Restaurants use microwaves and consuming items prepared in a microwave is a "no-no". There is nothing beneficial about microwave food other than it is quickly prepared and the results you get after heating or cooking food in a microwave are not welcome in the *Spiritual Royal* body.

High sodium content is another issue with restaurant food and all prepared foods. Adding an overabundance of salt or sugar seems to be the common practice in order to "add flavor". You will learn how to use fresh herbs, garlic and homemade broths for flavor.

THE WINDING ROAD

Some foods loose their negative effect when they are cooked down into a broth and strained out or mixed in a batter. This gives rise to the thought of whether it is the texture of the food, the fact it is raw, or any number of other reasons, and that maybe on its own it becomes stuck during its travels through the winding road of the intestines.

Onions, celery and eggs are three foods I have found to be troublesome on their own. Onions and celery I have cooked with other vegetables to make a broth and the broth has given me no issues. I strain the broth before use in a soup. Eggs are another troublesome character. Eggs alone, fried, scrambled or whatever form, produce a withdrawal to the Wheel bank account. Given that, I have used eggs in the fresh bread I make and in pancake batter and have done well with both. Maybe eggs need an escort to complete the journey through the winding path of intestines. Some foods just do not like to travel alone.

When baking, an alternative for eggs is 1 tablespoon of flax meal soaked in 3 tablespoons of water for about 5 minutes to replace one egg.

MYSTERIES OF FOODS

I Corinthians 8:8: *Food will not make us acceptable to God. We are not inferior if we don't eat, and we are not better if we do eat.* (HCS)

Foods are not going to change a level of power/energy God may decide to gift to a person or how God chooses to relate to a person. There is an underlying genetic factor that comes through a gentle whisper in this verse. (See also, I John 5:6-8).

Foods provide an avenue for the cells to be come clean, the Wheels to be properly charged and the body to live healthy. Food provides an important step to becoming a potential substation for power that would come through/ from the main power station (God). (See description of *Heaven Energy* under Terms.)

John 6:62-64: *Then what if you were to observe the Son of Man ascending to where He was before? The Spirit is the One that gives life. The flesh doesn't help at all. The words that I have spoken to you are spirit and are life. But there are some among you who don't believe.* (HCS)

DEATH OF ADDED SALT

Added salt had to be completely eliminated from my plate (including soy sauce and all condiments with high sodium content). Yes, we've all heard salt is a must for the body. While I am not a medical practitioner, I would invite the curious minds to review articles on lactate or lactic acid.

There is a process that takes place in the body when it breaks down glucose in the blood that could just quite possibly be what is being interfered with when there is too much salt in use. Can the body produce it's own salt? Sweat and tears are salty right? Babies don't eat salt and they have salty sweat and tears. If the proper form of glucose, through fruits not granulated sugars or corn syrups, is in the blood it is highly likely (I'm speaking from my own personal experiences here) the body converts that fruit-originated glucose into the salt the body needs. When salt is added in abundance, that natural process of glucose conversion is interrupted and, here I go again with no proof just thought processing, could result in issues with the pancreas, i.e., diabetes or pancreatic pains and inflammation. This may all shed a little light on obesity as well. When the glucose in the blood is not broken down and processed into the salt necessary for the body because the salt we added to our food took over it's role, wouldn't the glucose that doesn't pass through the kidneys end up stored within the body?

Another interesting detail I experienced is when I would wake up in the night and not have the ability to fall right back to sleep eventually I would end up hungry. As I lay awake I would wonder what it could have been that I encountered that day that would prevent my desired and necessary slumber. Having checked off all of the published possibilities (TV, computers, cell phones, climate in the bedroom, etc.) the idea of getting up to eat a bite or two of banana seemed to be the recurring theme. I would get up and eat a half of a banana, wash it down with a sip of water and return to bed and fall asleep within a few minutes. Once I caught on to what my body was telling me the remedy seemed quite simple. This happened repeated times. No, blood sugar levels were never an issue. There was something about the banana, possibly its high potassium content, that seemed to assist my body in processing the salt I had eaten that day which had triggered the interruption in my sleep.

Hopefully someone who has the ability to test these things can come forth in the future with insight or an equation of proof on the subject. You cannot argue with the fact that the banana was an inexpensive and simple remedy.

GRAINS

When the Wheels are charged and working properly, any issues with digesting grain will cease. Organic grains are always best but not always available. Whole grain, nothing fortified or enriched, has the nutrients you need when it has not been overly processed. Multigrain and seed breads have good flavor and make a tasty veggie sandwich with a little melted butter and some grated horseradish as a replacement for the usual condiment.

In the story of Pharaoh, grain was stored up for the coming famine. Contrary to many diet recommendations, grain is a benefit when prepared properly. Whole organic sprouted grains are the easiest to digest. This is coming from someone who had digestive disturbances for years and ate a gluten free diet before many people, including restaurants, even knew what the word gluten meant. There are nutrients in grain the body needs and, here's the glucose thoughts again, can assist in the process necessary for the production of salt in the body. Who was that that said carbs were bad?

Grain becomes hard to digest when there are underlying issues within the digestive system (parasites or Candida infections). It requires a dose of the *Heaven Energy* within the body to have the ability to break grains (gluten) down and process it without discomfort. Those issues must be addressed and corrected, and they will correct given the proper time. Charging up the Wheels for the digestive system will assist in recovery of the digestion.

There is no set period of time on any of the required steps toward optimum wellness because each person has a different degree of correction that must be made. When eating strictly fruits and vegetables the body will drop weight at a steady pace. Grain is your weight stabilizer.

Whole steel cut oats are beneficial, but not rolled oats. Cooking whole steel cut oats in apple juice (or other permissible juice) with a little butter and cinnamon or pumpkin pie spice is yummy and avoids the need of adding any sweetener. A brief list of food options will be at the back of the book.

Matthew 12:1: *At that time Jesus passed through the grain fields on the Sabbath. His disciples were hungry and began to pick and eat some heads of grain.* (HCS)

MEATS AND FISH

Ezekiel 28:22-23: *Look! I am against you Sidon and I will display My glory within (among) you. They will know that I am Yahweh when I execute judgments against her and demonstrate My holiness through her. I will send a plague against her and bloodshed in her streets; the slain will fall within her, while the sword is against her on every side. Then they will know that I am Yahweh.* (HCS)(Emphasis added)

Sidon: To hunt or fish; to get meat rather than veggies; hunting game; net or stronghold; provisions of food. [Arabim-publications.com]

Ezekiel speaks of the judgment of God coming against those who choose to eat meats or fish over vegetables. In other words, there are consequences to the physical body that will take place when meat or fish are the food of choice. A *Spiritual Royal* will not function well on meats or fish, various symptoms eventually manifest when eating a meat, including poultry, and fish diet. There may be various reasons for this and having walked through a time in life where meat was a food choice for me, I can speak from experience on how the body will feel and its ability to recover when meat is eliminated from the diet.

Red meats contain the blood that has record of its life

experiences by means of vibration or frequencies. Those frequencies likely cause interference with the human cells (our blood record). Here's something to consider: If our blood cells can record what our ancestors ate or the emotions they had, wouldn't it make sense that the blood of animals can do the same thing? Why wouldn't the blood of the animal have record of their life experiences of extreme weather conditions or being chased by a tiger or any number of other experiences an animal may have. Then when we eat that animal with the blood aren't we consuming those blood frequencies of the animal? Maybe this is one reason why Scripture, God specifically, tells us to avoid eating the meats. A mystery held in the hands of God alone. Scripture does not expand on the 'why', it just states eating meat and fish will result in a "plague" (health issues).

A warning is given to those who hunt and fish as a means for food. For hundreds of years many people gathered meat and fish as a source of food for survival reasons. Scripture is advising against this and Ezekiel is not the only place this avoidance of meat products is addressed. There can be multiple reasons "why" people began eating flesh products even when it was advised against. First, as mentioned above, lack of other sources of food.

In the winter it is challenging, if not impossible dependent upon where you live, to grow fresh food in a garden. Short of owning a green house it can be impossible. As people scattered to various areas around the world their food source changed. When a person eats a specific diet (i.e., meats) over an extended period of time and that same diet is carried out over generations, the body (and blood) becomes encoded with the notion that meat is the food source and that 'meat code' passes through to the next generation. It is as though the body becomes programmed to eat meat and limited plant sources. The body (through cell messages) tells the individual where the relief from hunger came from via their ancestral genetic imprints.

People who lived by a clean water source ate fish so the generations after that initial survival act of eating just fish took place, the descendants hunger for fish. Until those preprogrammed messages are changed, the body will tell you it wants fish (or meat). Itchy or dry flaky skin can be a result of eating fish or fish oils.

Genesis 9:3-5: *Every moving thing that liveth shall be meat for you; even as the green herb have I given you all things. But flesh with the life thereof, which is the blood thereof, shall ye not eat. And surely your blood of your lives will I require; at the hand of every beast will I require it, and at the hand of man; at the hand of every man's brother will I require the life of man.* (KJV) (Emphasis added)

I'm going to suggest that the reference to "every moving thing" in Genesis means everything that is moved by growth or the wind and not a reference to the creatures with feet or wings, simply because the following sentence tell us to stay away from flesh with the blood (life). Flesh with the life in it (blood) is not to be eaten or your own blood/body will pay a price. God has issued a protective order over animals by stating that at the 'hand of every beast' (on behalf of) He will require a payback. That payback is seen today in blood tests that reflect such things as heart disease, high cholesterol, etc.

Ezekiel 23:38: *They also did this to Me: they defiled My sanctuary on that same day and profaned My Sabbaths.* (HCS)

Ezekiel 44:7: *When you brought in foreigners, uncircumcised in both heart and flesh, to occupy My sanctuary, you defiled My temple while you offered My food – the fat and the blood. You broke My covenant by all your detestable practices.* (HCS)

II Corinthians 12:7-9: *And lest I should be exalted above measure through the abundance of the revelations, there was given to me a thorn in the flesh, the messenger of Satan to buffet me, lest I should be exalted above measure. For this thing I besought the Lord thrice, that it might depart from me. And he said unto me, My grace is sufficient for thee; for my strength is made perfect in weakness. Most gladly therefore will I rather glory in my infirmities, that the power of Christ may rest upon me.* (KJV)

The thorn referenced in II Corinthians is something that is bothersome. Keeping on the track of genetics or blood, it can be viewed as an act of the cells that tell you to want some form of food a *Spiritual Royal* is not to have; something that would "kill, steal and destroy" (aka Satan) your life. That nagging reminder of how tasty the french fries or chocolate ice cream was.

People are not perfect and are not designed to be perfect, that's God's job. In order to keep people out of the perfect category, we will at times step out of the boundary lines of the food restrictions, described as "weakness" in II Corinthians. This keeps us human. God extends a grace, or padding in that health bank account I referenced previously, where we will not plummet instantly into a state of disease. Getting back on the right track is key.

I Corinthians 8:13: *Therefore, if food causes my brother to fall, I will never again eat meat, so that I won't cause my brother to fall.* (HCS)

POULTRY

I have not found chicken or turkey to be beneficial. Chicken has more of a neutral affect and turkey has been a negative food. To avoid potential argument over the point of avoiding poultry as a consumable food, let's look at Numbers 11.

Numbers 11:31-32: *And there went forth a wind from the Lord, and brought quails from the sea, and let them fall by the camp, as it were a day's journey on this side, and as it were a day's journey on the other side, round about the camp and as it were two cubits high upon the face of the earth. And the people stood up all that day, and all that night, and all the next day, and they gathered the quails; he that gathered least gathered ten homers; and they spread them all abroad for themselves around the camp.* (KJV)

Psalm 105:40: *The people asked, and he brought quails, and satisfied them with the bread of heaven.* (KJV)

Many times the reference to an animal in Scripture is symbolic of some form of characteristic or protective or destructive element. Quails in Scripture appear to represent a form of protection. Psalm 105 speaks of a wide spread (not personal) means of support for the livelihood of the people. Quails were used in the Middle Ages as

a form of protection from lightning strikes (thesymbolism.
com). The reference to the quail being gathered from the
sea and the fact that quail do not live in or above the sea,
could be an indication of a storm connection here; storms
often originate over seas/oceans.

GOT MILK?

Proverbs 27:27: *And thou shalt have goats' milk enough for thy food, for the food of thy household, and for the maintenance for thy maidens.* (KJV)

Hebrews 5:13: *For every one that useth milk is unskillful in the word of righteousness for he is a babe.* (KJV)

Coming from a family that has numerous members that have experienced struggles with digesting milk and milk products, goat's milk became the go-to at times for the babies.

I read an article years ago and do not recall where I read it, that the molecular structure or particles of goat's milk is similar to that of human milk. With the Scripture above referencing "maintenance for the maidens", we can safely apply that this is speaking of those who helped care for the babies when the birth mother couldn't. If a birth mother was unable to feed her newborn for whatever reasons, the maidens were there to take their place and would either nurse the baby themselves or use goat's milk as the replacement. The same would ring true for today, a replacement for breast milk for an infant should be goat's milk to achieve an ease in the digestive process. No more crying babies makes a momma happy.

Cow's milk causes a deduction in the Wheel and cell bank account and in addition can be littered with stress hormones from the milking process, hormones given to the cow to increase milk production and other chemicals used for the "health" of the milk cow. There are only two cow's milk products I have found to not cause a deduction in the health bank account and they are: organic, grass fed, unsalted cow's butter and organic Bulgarian yogurt, no sugars, no flavors. Try to find a local source when possible.

There are many other options available for milk replacement such as nut milks. Keep in mind these milks often have additives in them, such as sunflower lecithin and salt. While the milk replacements may work for a milk replacement in cooking, I never found them beneficial over an extended period of time. Extended use seemed to deplete the Wheel and cell health bank account.

HERBS

Genesis 1:29-30: *And God said, Behold I have given you every herb bearing seed, which is upon the face of all the earth, and every tree in the which is the fruit of a tree yielding seed; to you it shall be for meat. And to every beast of the earth and every fowl of the air, and to every thing that creepeth upon the earth, wherein there is life, I have given every green herb for meat and it was so.* (KJV)

Genesis 47:24: *And it shall come to pass in the increase, that ye shall give the fifth part unto Pharaoh, and four parts shall be your own, for seed of the field, and for your food, and for them of your households, and for food for your little ones.* (KJV)

Ezekiel 47:12: *And by the river upon the bank thereof, on this side and on that side, shall grow all trees for meat, whose leaf shall not fade, neither shall the fruit thereof be consumed: it shall bring forth new fruit according to his months, because their waters they issued out of the sanctuary and the fruit thereof shall be for meat, and the leaf thereof for medicine.* (KJV)

Seed of the field tells us to look to plants for sustenance; seed is provided to keep the cycle of food production going. There are numerous herbs available in various forms.

47

In Ezekiel 47 there is a reference to the leaves being used for medicines. Herbal supplements are available through practitioners or local health food stores and can be used for numerous discomforts. Consult a qualified practitioner and use quality herbs for any attempt to correct an issue inside the body.

Herbs are also available in the form of essential oils and can be quite beneficial. Again, consult a handbook written by a professional before use for any health disturbance. For casual use, I use essential oils daily.

MAYBE MONEY DOES GROW ON TREES

Leviticus 19:23-26: *And when ye shall come into the land, and shall have planted all manner of trees for food, then ye shall count the fruit thereof as uncircumcised; three years shall it be as uncircumcised unto you; it shall not be eaten of. But in the fourth year all the fruit thereof shall be holy to praise the Lord withal. And in the fifth year shall ye eat of the fruit thereof, that it may yield unto you the increase thereof; I am the Lord your God. Ye shall not eat anything with the blood; neither shall ye use enchantment nor observe times.* (KJV)

There are restrictions for consuming fruit (produce) from any tree until the fifth year of growth. The tree must be allowed to mature to a certain point before the fruit is acceptable or beneficial for consumption. If there are any orchard owners (or those who desire to start an orchard) within the sound of my voice, this is vital information for you. The trees are not to be used for profit or their fruit for consumption until the fifth year.

Today, the consumer has no way of knowing how old a tree is before the producers of that particular fruit pick it and sell it to a grocery store. There must be a component to the affects the fruit would have on the body energetically for such a reference to be put in Scripture.

Let the trees have their time of maturing and God will bless your crops; fall outside the lines of instruction given in Scripture and the life of your orchard may struggle. God's eyes scan the whole earth.

CITRUS

Other than lemon juice from a fresh lemon, citrus is not friendly to the cell health bank account either. I do not know the history of where oranges, grapefruits, limes, etc. began but something about them simply does not add up to a good deposit into the health bank account.

We've all heard how that glass of orange juice is a must for your vitamin C intake but any proof of benefit was not taken to the level of inside the cells. Vitamin C is available in many fruits and vegetables, not just oranges. Makes you wonder if there is a deeper message to the orange groves (orchards) struggling as a result of the cooler weather. Sometimes God sends messages we just haven't picked up on yet.

Citrus in the form of essential oils are great for disinfecting or general household cleaning.

NUTS AND SEEDS

Nuts have a reputation of containing mold. I settled for purchasing organic raw almonds that I would soak in water over night in order to sprout them, remove the skins and then dry the almonds in the convection oven the next day. I store them in the freezer to avoid any possible onset of mold.

Organic raw almond butter has served many purposes and proved no harm. Peanuts and peanut butter on the other hand tip the scales the opposite direction. Having read up on molds in the past, some nut varieties carry mold in the folds of the meat of the nut. Walnuts were the worst according to the report; pecans can have mold as well. I have used cashews and almonds in recipes and have not experienced any negative response. Some of the new paleo products are made with cashews and I have tried a few of those. Treeline makes a plant based French style cheese spread that I have used with cassava tortillas.

Eat seeds in abundance if you like. Organic sunflower seeds I soak to sprout and dry in the convection oven. These are much easier than a nut to get completely dry so I store them in a glass container. I use sunflower seeds in nearly everything. Pumpkin seeds, chia seeds and sesame seeds are beneficial as well. They contain a good source of beneficial oils for the body and add a little crunch to your salad.

Seed butters are permissible as long as they don't contain sugar or other additives. To date I have not found a sprouted seed butter.

OH HOW SWEET

No sugars, other than maple syrup or honey, if necessary. Refined sugars, cane sugar and corn syrups lack life and will deplete your cell health bank account. My personal journey has revealed pure maple syrup (not flavored corn syrup) is beneficial; honey is not harmful but should be eaten sparingly.

I do not know if it is the fact that most refined sugars come from the cane sugar plant which is from the grass family or what the specifics are that cause it to be harmful; coconut sugar is another sweetener that does not register as a beneficial option, nor does the flesh of a coconut. Coconut oils have their benefits when applied directly to the skin or hair but don't seem to jive with the interior of the body.

Fresh fruits have proven time and again to be the best option for adding a little sweet into the diet.

SERIOUSLY? NO CAFFEINE OR CHOCOLATE?

No caffeine, it acts as a diuretic and results in dehydrating the body of the fluids it needs to flush out toxic components from the cells. Locking harmful imprints into the cells opens the opportunity for cancers. In order to shift the interior of the cells, all caffeine will need to be avoided. It acts like a jail cell preventing release of the very things you need to get rid of. Coffee, like teas, have mold. That morning cup of java may in fact be "defiling your temple."

Jeremiah 7:30: *For the Judeans have done what is evil in My sight. This is the Lord's declaration. "They have set up their detestable things in the house that is called by My name and defiled it."* (HCS) (That "house" is your body.)

Psalm 79:1: *God, the nations have invaded Your inheritance, desecrated Your holy temple, and turned Jerusalem into ruins.* (HCS) (This verse is talking about a specific people group (Judeans/Israelites), the inside of their body and how it no longer resides in peace (Jerusalem)).

Yes, this includes the cocoa bean; chocolate is very acidic and is harmful as well. I know, I've heard the reports too about how good it is for you. Remember, the tests on the products we hear about are often times not run through all available testing, or full disclosure of any test is lacking.

They test in order to obtain an avenue for sales. I doubt that any product to date has been tested on the benefit/harm it may produce inside the cells, or if it hinders cell receptor sites.

I have yet to find a replacement for chocolate although I have found chicory root to be a replacement for coffee. It's easy to brew and when you add a cinnamon stick or cardamom seed while it is brewing it does the trick. Chicory is caffeine free and provides alkaline to the system. The alkaline aids in easing the discomfort of acid reflux and will help keep the pH balanced versus coffee that can cause an acidic upset and moves the pH toward acidic.

Ezekiel 5:11: *Therefore, as I live – this is the declaration of the Lord God – "I am going to cut you off and show you no pity, because you have defiled My sanctuary with all your detestable practices and abominations. Yes, I will not spare you."* (HCS)

FLAVORINGS

There are reports of laboratory proof that red food coloring has health consequences for certain individuals. I will add to this and say flavorings of all types can interfere with something that has to do with the neurotransmitters, or brain electrical activity. This would include all those added artificial or natural cherry, mint, coffee, etc. flavors seen on the labels of waters, sodas, syrups, coffees and many packaged foods, which are off the table for a *Spiritual Royal* anyway. If you need to add a flavor to something, use a good quality spice or fresh herb.

WATER IS YOUR NEW BEST FRIEND

There are numerous types of water available these days and every company thinks theirs is the best. City tap water is not an acceptable option when you are walking through the process of cleaning out debris from the cells. Reverse Osmosis water has withstood the tests I gave it, along with a few of the alkaline waters. A diet heavy in coffee, chocolate or meat will result in being acidic and will need to be addressed by taking steps to balance the pH level in the body. Two ways I have found to address acidic pH is with alkaline water and potassium supplements. Both inexpensive and have given me no negative kickback.

To boost the benefit of your water of choice, use a tuning fork, strike it and hold it over the glass of water for a few seconds, or hold the end of the tuning fork against the glass. This vibration will record into the water molecules elevating the benefit of the water.

HERBAL TEAS

Scripture describes defilement being from various forms, including mold. Scripture directs attention to the interior of a building versus the interior of the body. Those references to structural buildings in an interpretation for today point to the interior of the physical body; our body is the temple (I Corinthians 6:19).

We have already eliminated any form of caffeine, which includes the typical black and green tea selections but we need to add caution to herbal teas as well. Teas often contain mold. The tea I found most harmful was peppermint and there are possibly many others. Marketed for its ability to aid digestion, I discovered it was creating an entire new set of problems. I have received benefit from organic Rooibos tea. Outside of that, I resorted to hot water with fresh cut or graded ginger and a splash of fresh lemon juice.

PROCESSED FOODS

As you have probably guessed by now, there are no processed foods that are a benefit. Many contain salt or sugar and other additives that simply do not help with recharging the Wheels and cause more of a reduction than a benefit.

ONE BAD APPLE

Foods can trigger E-motions. When food is eaten during a period of extreme or extended E-motion, the food consumed during those times can become a trigger for a repeat of the E-motion(s). Example: During a time of grief the individual eats macaroni and cheese. Months or even years later, eating pasta, cheese or macaroni and cheese can remind the body of the prior grief E-motion, causing the individual to feel the grief all over again.

There is a hidden communication that takes place between the body (specifically cells) and food. The body is a very complex machine and is much more sensitive than once thought.

1 Samuel 14:24: *And the men of Israel were distressed that day: for Saul had adjured the people, saying, Cursed be the man that eateth any food until evening, that I may be avenged on mine enemies. So none of the people tasted any food. (KJV)*

KEEP ON THE MOVE

It is challenging to erase the images that have become connected to a private gym or community recreation center when using the word exercise. When I reference exercise, I am not referring to any form of strenuous, muscle building or toning form of movement, which can actually put a strain on the interior functions the body. A more appropriate description for what is <u>beneficial</u> for the physical body is "remain active".

To be active can encompass many things and is certainly less expensive than a membership fee at a gym. COVID ushered in the opportunity for individuals to begin exercising within their own home, which is a move in a beneficial direction. I never wanted to go and share sweat with a bunch of people, especially those I did not know, and never had challenges with my weight other than being under weight while going through the transitions necessary for cleaning out the cells. Any blood work I ever had would reflect I was "exercising" and that resulted in being questioned what type of exercise I did. Under a standard category of "exercise" I did none. I stay active.

By active I mean things such as: having a vegetable garden or flower garden; walks or hikes in nature; a leisurely bike ride; occasional snow skiing; cleaning house (laundry, dishes, sweeping, mopping, vacuuming, all things a surgeon will tell you to avoid after you have a surgery so they must have some beneficial muscle toning component); and stretching.

When your body is free of the cell debris, it knows how to remain strong and will not need specific toning style exercises. It is when an individual becomes sedentary (and over loaded with toxic cells) that the muscles begin to decline, cellulite sets in and strength fades away.

Running or doing strengthening exercises until the muscles are rock hard cannot be a benefit to the electrical activity that must go on in the body, not to mention the fact that the more exercise of that category is done the more likely the heart muscle is hardening up as well. I have not found a reference in Scripture that states Jesus, His disciples, or any other prominent character in the Bible, jogged or ran anywhere. Yes, physical labor existed and people walked or hiked many miles; they were active. They did not over exert their physical bodies with the intent of obtaining a response other than becoming tired. If a person was a slave, they may have been forced to over exert but that was not a choice of their own nor for seeking a result of change to the physical body.

Today, many people sit at a desk most of the day and need some form of daily physical movement. My suggestion is get up from the desk every hour or so and go for a short walk, stretch the legs a bit. Sitting all day and then going on a 3 mile run or participating in strenuous exercise cannot be good for the body; there's too many extremes involved in that sort of schedule. Balance in all things is important; moderation is key or you tip the scales.

During my journey I put 2-and-2 together that any form of activity that puts the head in a position below the waist (bending over) or a headstand style position is not natural and reaps little, if any, benefit. After an extended period of time my inverted exercises began to make my eardrums feel as though they were pulsing. God only knows what else it may have been doing to my head! Sure, placing the head in a position toward the floor while the rest of the body is elevated above it will push blood circulation toward the head but why is that necessary? Do we not think God knew what he was doing when He put our head at the top of the body with no feet on it? If we needed more blood to get to our brain He would have added more avenues for blood to get there.

CLOTHING

As odd as it may be to some, the fabric your clothing and bedding is made from can interfere with or be an asset to the electrical activity within you and around you.

Our body receives energy waves from the planets, moon and stars. If you cover yourself in fabrics that deny those energy waves to get to you, it can hinder your ability to recharge the Wheels, make strides in purging toxins from the cells and interfere with the ability to gain proper rest and recovery for the body.

Organic materials are best but often can be quite costly. When it comes to replacing all those manufactured materials, start with small changes and advance through time. Linen, wool, cotton, alpaca and bamboo fabrics have all been beneficial.

POWER OF THE TONGUE

Oh, be careful little mouth, or in some cases big mouth, what you say! Words hold power and can deplete the Wheel health bank account. All of those beneficial foods you ate during the day quite possibly could lose their good benefit if the tongue is giving off a display of curses or gossip rather than blessing.

Proverbs 18:21: *Life and death are in the power of the tongue, and those who love it will eat its fruit.* (HCS)

SPIRIT FOOD vs. FLESH FOOD

I selected the title of "Spirit Food" to reflect the foods that feed life (or energy) into the body and cells; the foods that if held under a black light would shine with vibrant color.

"Flesh Food" was selected to reference food that will pass through the digestive system with seemingly little or no issues but does not provide an energetic deposit into the health bank account.

Spirit Foods

Dairy
Bulgarian Yogurt (no sugar, no flavor)
Butter (grass fed, no salt)
Ghee
Mozzarella Cheese

Fruits
Apple
Avocado
Banana
Berries (Black, Blue, Raspberry,
Strawberry)
Dark Cherries
Melon (Cantaloupe, Honey Dew,
Watermelon)
Pear
Pineapple
Tomato

Grains
Amaranth
Brown Rice
Corn meal
Millet
Oats (steel cut/whole)

Quinoa
Whole Sprouted Wheat (no fortified)

All fresh Herbs

Jelly and Juices
Big B's Apples juices (apple; apple cherry,
apple ginger; apple pear)
Lemon juice, fresh
Pineapple Juice (organic, no sugars)
St. Dalfour Fruit Spreads

Nuts
Almond (raw, sprouted)
Almond Butter
Brazil
Cashew

Oils/Fat
Avocado Oil
Butter (organic, no salt, grass fed cow's)
Ghee
Sunflower Oil

Other
Alkaline Water
Cassava Tortillas
Chicory Root
Ginger Root
Honey (raw, organic)

Maple Syrup (pure; it also comes in
granulated form)
Treeline Cashew spreads

Seeds
Chia
Flax meal
Poppy
Pumpkin
Sesame
Sunflower

Vegetables
Artichoke
Baby Bok Choy
Baby Broccoli
Beets
Brussel Sprouts
Butternut Squash
Carrot
Cucumber
Green Bean
Green Peas
Horseradish
Kale
Lettuce (all, minus iceberg)
Mushrooms (White or Baby Bella)
Pumpkin
Radish
Red Bell Pepper
Spinach

Sugar Snap Peas
Sweet Potato (and yam)
Swiss Chard
Zucchini

Flesh Foods

Beans
No bean has been found to be a benefit

Dairy
Blue Cheese (and most other cheese)
Milk (Cow's)
Eggs

Fruits
Citrus

Grains
Kernel Corn

All meats, poultry and fish

Other
Apple Cider Vinegar
Anything with added sugar
Chocolate; Cacao
Coconut
Coffee
Condiments and Dressings
Olive Oil
Pickles

Processed Foods
Salt
Soy Sauce
Teas, black, green and most herbal

Vegetable
Asparagus
Cabbage
Cauliflower
Celery
Ice Berg Lettuce
Onions
Potato (white, yellow, red skin)

TERMS

<u>Frequencies/Vibration</u> terms are used to direct attention to the activity inside cells or the unseen response to a source of energy. Most of what is referenced in this book will be the toxic or harmful frequencies that develop into physical symptoms (headaches, skin irritations, joint aches, etc.) and can eventually turn into disease (heart disease, cancers, etc.). I do not use technical medical terms 1) because I'm not overly familiar with them; 2) so the general population can get a better understanding of the message I am attempting to relay. A good visual when you see the term frequency or vibration is static that would come over a radio or weakness in the sound waves it is attempting to transmit.

<u>Heaven Energy</u> is the term selected to reference the invisible, powerful, potentially life altering force(s) that reside in the Heavens or Firmament and Universe and have an influence on the atmosphere in which we live and the physical body we occupy. Heaven Energy is the main power station; our physical body can be a substation for the power station to distribute its energy to and through, when the substation is structurally sound and in optimum working order.

Spiritual Royal is the term selected to describe the genetic inheritance of or genetic advancement toward cells within the body that contain an advanced level of electrical charge (often referred to as "Spirit" in Scripture). The evidence of any Spiritual Gift (elevated charge within the cells or other electrical conduction in the body) will unfold through what is called the "royal priesthood" in Scripture. *Spiritual Royals* have what I call Star Dust (advanced level of electrical conduction) in their blood.

Wheels are the electrical centers that run along the spine. Think of them like small rechargeable battery packs. The Wheels are referenced in the book of Ezekiel. Wheels are called chakras in the Sanskrit language. In order to follow Scripture more easily and to create a new identity outside of what is common in Indian culture, the name Wheel(s) will be used.

God placed Adam and Eve
in a Garden,
not in a pasture.

Resources

Arabim-publications.com
Holy Bible (King James Version; Holman
        Christian Standard)
Life
Thesymbolism.com

www.ingramcontent.com/pod-product-compliance
Lightning Source LLC
Chambersburg PA
CBHW031549260326
41914CB00002B/334